Published by First Place 4 Health
Houston, Texas
www.firstplace4health.com
Printed in the U.S.A.

© 2014, 2008 First Place 4 Health.
All rights reserved.

ISBN 978-1-942425-06-9

All Scripture quotations are taken from the *Holy Bible, New International Version®*, NIV®
Copyright © 1973, 1978, 1984, 2011 by Biblica, Inc. Used by permission of Zondervan.
All rights reserved worldwide. www.zondervan.com The "NIV" and "New International
Version" are trademarks registered in the United States Patent and Trademark Office by Biblica, Inc.
NASB—Scripture taken from the *New American Standard Bible,*

the value of prayer journals

Believing that God wants His children to pray, I began writing my prayers in April 1990. For several years, I had resisted praying in this manner. Being a fun-loving individual, I felt that writing my prayers would be time consuming, to say the least. At that time, my prayer life was not something I found pleasant or rewarding. I felt five minutes was a long time to pray. My thoughts would begin to wander and before I knew it, I was planning the day ahead, rather than praying. I had attended seminars on prayer for years. I thought some secret formula must exist that would make me a mighty prayer warrior. That is until I began prayer journaling.

The greatest benefit I have received from writing my prayers is the total focus on praying while I am writing. My mind is focused because it is difficult to write and think of other things at the same time. Also, the Holy Spirit directs my praying when my mind is tuned in to God. My faith grows tremendously as I go back through my journal and highlight the many answers to prayer in my life.

God has taught me many truths through journaling. I have learned to praise Him in all things. Trials in my life may seem like roadblocks to me, but God sees these trials as stepping-stones to victory and spiritual growth. Journaling has taught me that God hears and answers all my prayers. When I pray within the framework of God's will, His answer is always a resounding yes! When God tells me no, He does so because I have asked something contrary to His will for my life. Many times what I perceive as His "No" is only "Wait, my child—the timing is not yet right."

Because of what God can do in your life, I recommend that you begin writing your thoughts and prayers. This journal is designed to assist you. My prayer is that God will use this process to help you focus your attention on Him as you pray. God bless you as you begin to fill this spiritual journey.

—*Carole Lewis*

Seek first his kingdom and his righteousness,
and all these things will be given to you as well.

MATTHEW 6:33

spiritual

emotional   physical

mental

spiritual

emotional

physical

mental

spiritual

emotional

physical

mental

spiritual

emotional

physical

mental

If you believe, you will receive whatever
you ask for in prayer.

MATTHEW 21:22

spiritual

emotional physical

mental

spiritual

emotional

physical

mental

spiritual

emotional　physical

mental

spiritual

emotional

physical

mental

Whoever has my commands and obeys them, he is the one who loves me.
He who loves me will be loved by my Father, and I too will love him and show myself to him.

JOHN 14:21

spiritual

emotional

physical

mental

spiritual

emotional

physical

mental

spiritual

emotional

physical

mental

spiritual

physical

emotional

mental

You know my folly, O God;
my guilt is not hidden from you.

PSALM 69:5

spiritual

emotional

physical

mental

spiritual

emotional

physical

mental

spiritual

emotional

physical

mental

spiritual

emotional

physical

mental

No temptation has seized you except what is common to man. And God is faithful, he will not let you be tempted beyond what you can bear. But when you are tempted, he will also provide a way out so that you can stand up under it.

1 CORINTHIANS 10:13

spiritual

emotional

physical

mental

spiritual

emotional

physical

mental

spiritual

emotional

physical

mental

spiritual

emotional

physical

mental

Man does not live on bread alone,
but on every word that comes from the mouth of God.

MATTHEW 4:4

spiritual

emotional

physical

mental

spiritual

emotional

physical

mental

spiritual

emotional

physical

mental

spiritual

emotional physical

mental

Do not conform any longer to the pattern of this world, but be transformed by the renewing of your mind. Then you will be able to test and approve what God's will is—his good, pleasing and perfect will.

ROMANS 12:2

spiritual

emotional

physical

mental

spiritual

emotional

physical

mental

spiritual

emotional

physical

mental

spiritual

emotional

physical

mental

Do you not know that your body is a temple of the Holy Spirit, who is in you, whom you have received from God? You are not your own; you were bought at a price. Therefore honor God with your body.

1 CORINTHIANS 6:19-20

spiritual

emotional physical

mental

spiritual

emotional

physical

mental

spiritual

emotional

physical

mental

spiritual

emotional physical

mental

Commit to the Lord whatever you do,
and your plans will succeed.

PROVERBS 16:3

spiritual

emotional

physical

mental

spiritual

emotional

physical

mental

spiritual

emotional

physical

mental

spiritual

emotional physical

mental

A new command I give you: Love one another. As I have loved you, so you must love one another. By this all men will know that you are my disciples, if you love one another.

JOHN 13:34-35

spiritual

emotional physical

mental

spiritual

emotional

physical

mental

spiritual

emotional

physical

mental

spiritual
emotional
physical
mental

I press on toward the goal to win the prize for which
God has called me heavenward in Christ Jesus.

PHILIPPIANS 3:14

spiritual

emotional physical

mental

spiritual

emotional

physical

mental

spiritual

emotional

physical

mental

spiritual

emotional

physical

mental

By faith Abraham, when called to go to a place he would later receive as his inheritance, obeyed and went, even though he did not know where he was going.

Hebrews 11:8

spiritual

emotional physical

mental

spiritual

emotional

physical

mental

spiritual

emotional

physical

mental

spiritual

emotional

physical

mental

But the worries of this life, the deceitfulness of wealth and the desires
for other things come in and choke the word, making it unfruitful.

MARK 4:19

spiritual

emotional

physical

mental

spiritual

emotional   physical

mental

spiritual

emotional

physical

mental

spiritual

emotional

physical

mental

And over all these virtues put on love,
which binds them all together in perfect unity.

COLOSSIANS 3:14

spiritual

emotional

physical

mental

spiritual

emotional

physical

mental

spiritual

emotional

physical

mental

spiritual

emotional

physical

mental

But you, man of God, flee from all this, and pursue righteousness,
godliness, faith, love, endurance and gentleness.

1 TIMOTHY 6:11

spiritual

emotional

physical

mental

spiritual

emotional

physical

mental

spiritual

emotional

physical

mental

spiritual

emotional

physical

mental

Do you not know that in a race all the runners run, but only one gets the prize?
Run in such a way as to get the prize.

1 CORINTHIANS 9:24

spiritual

emotional

physical

mental

spiritual

emotional

physical

mental

spiritual

emotional

physical

mental

spiritual

emotional   physical

mental

When the Chief Shepherd appears,
you will receive the crown of glory that will never fade away.

1 Peter 5:4

spiritual

emotional

physical

mental

spiritual

emotional

physical

mental

spiritual

emotional

physical

mental

spiritual

physical

mental

emotional

Therefore, since we are surrounded by such a great cloud of witnesses, let us throw off everything that hinders and the sin that so easily entangles, and let us run with perseverance the race marked out for us.

HEBREWS 12:1

spiritual

emotional physical

mental

spiritual

emotional   physical

mental

spiritual
emotional
physical
mental

spiritual

emotional

physical

mental

Let us fix our eyes on Jesus, the author and perfecter of our faith, who for the joy set before him endured the cross, scorning its shame, and sat down at the right hand of the throne of God.

HEBREWS 12:2

spiritual

emotional physical

mental

spiritual

emotional

physical

mental

spiritual

emotional

physical

mental

spiritual

emotional physical

mental

See to it that no one misses the grace of God and that no bitter root grows up to cause trouble and defile many.

HEBREWS 12:15

spiritual

emotional

physical

mental

spiritual

emotional

physical

mental

spiritual

emotional

physical

mental

spiritual

emotional

physical

mental

The LORD has done great things for us,
and we are filled with joy.

PSALM 126:3

spiritual

emotional

physical

mental